To Mylo,
God Bless You!
Sharon Hoffman
Prov. 31:30

The Today Girl

The Today Girl

Sharon Hoffman

Fleming H. Revell Company
Old Tappan, New Jersey

Scripture quotations in this volume are from the King James Version of the Bible.

No part of this book may be reproduced in any manner without written permission from the publisher, except for brief quotations embodied in critical articles and reviews. Total Girl classes may not be taught from this material. For information and permission to teach Total Girl classes, address Total Girl, 9350 Robinson Street Overland Park, Kansas 66212

Library of Congress Cataloging in Publication Data

Hoffman, Sharon.
   The today girl.

   SUMMARY: Presents a Christian approach to being a pleasing, feminine, and popular date and to preparing oneself to be a loving and giving wife.
    1. Dating (Social customs) 2. Girls—Conduct of life. 3. Interpersonal relations. 4. Sex instruction for girls. [1. Dating (Social customs) 2. Conduct of life] I. Title.
HQ801.H64   301.41'42   76–6077
ISBN 0-8007-0792-3

Copyright © 1976 by Fleming H. Revell Company
All Rights Reserved
Printed in the United States of America

TO my husband, Rob,
Whose love and understanding has made my life TOTAL.

Acknowledgments

TO *Marabel Morgan,* whose course on marriage and the family inspired these writings for single girls;

TO *Bobbie Evans,* for her initial inspiration and encouragement in making this book a reality;

TO *Pam McCord,* for her hours of prayerful assistance in polishing this manuscript;

TO *Rev. Larry Moff,* whose messages on marriage and the home inspired the outline for my final chapter;

AND TO *all the graduates of the* TOTAL GIRL *classes:* May their efforts be rewarded throughout their eventual marriages.

Contents

Foreword   11

1. **Me, Myself, and I**   17

   Smile! You Are Somebody
   Girl Friend or Mother-Image?
   Your Curb Appeal
   Snack-Snitchers
   Time to Spare
   Homework 1

2. **Securing His Attention**   37

   Right Place, Right Time
   Winning His Initial Interest
   The First Big Date
   Everybody's Not Doing It!
   Biblical Restraint
   Homework 2

3. **Creative Dating**   47

   Let's Celebrate
   Filling His Cup
   Crown Him King
   Mend His Wounds

Yes, Let's!
Forgive and Forget
Childlike Reactions
Asking and Receiving
Homework 3

4. Dating Seriously   65

Marriage Material—Him
G—Godly
I—Influence
R—Rich
L—Lovely
Homework 4

THE TEN QUALITIES OF TRUE LOVE   75

5. How to Measure the Quality of Your Love   77

Conclusion: The Today Girl Is the TOTAL GIRL   95

Foreword

Here is a book for YOU—to help you to be the teenage girl of TODAY, with all the exciting possibilities of developing your very own personality. Sharon Hoffman has the ability to communicate on a teen level—a skill she has perfected through her highly successful TOTAL GIRL courses. The warm, sincere, understanding atmosphere she creates readily wins the confidence and respect of her girls, enabling Mrs. Hoffman to provide Christian guidance for the teenager of today—and the Total Woman of tomorrow.

YOU—*The Today Girl*—are encouraged to make the most of your natural beauty and individual personality—to be feminine, in your own distinctive way. Mrs. Hoffman discusses dating frankly. Hints are provided for you to keep the dating sessions fun, and to show you how you can be the ideal dating partner. Sharon Hoffman points out that sex is for marriage, describing how you can avoid the pitfalls of a too-intimate relationship. She sets forth the Ten Qualities of True Love, explaining how you know "it's the real thing."

TOTAL GIRL: That's what you—*The Today Girl*—can become. And that's what the readers of this book will discover through the Christ-centered and practical insights of Sharon Hoffman.

THE PUBLISHERS

"I cannot do much," said a little star,
"To make the dark world bright;
My silver beams cannot travel far
Through the folding gloom of night.
But I'm only a part of God's great plan,
And I'll cheerfully do the best I can."

AUTHOR UNKNOWN

The
Today Girl

1

Me, Myself, and I!

"He's absolutely *the* neatest guy in our school, and I get to go to the game Saturday night with him."

"I know you must be about to die! I wouldn't be able to sleep or eat or do anything until Saturday night."

Sound familiar, girls? Some of the best times a teenage girl has are those chats with a close friend flopped over the bed in the privacy of her bedroom. Let's do just that. Move over your stuffed animals and make yourself comfortable for a time of casual conversation.

My own teenage years (about which I could write volumes) were mostly of hardship and heartbreak. Selfishly, I was out to get all the honors and all the fellows I could. Realizing that brought no satisfaction, I set out to find the solution to my disappointments. I found answers and began applying them to my way of life. What a change! My whole attitude turned around—toward my dress, speech, boys, and my whole outlook for the future. That's why I want to share these principles with you. They worked in my life, and I am seeing them work on other girls' lives even now.

Every girl that I've ever met wants to be liked, look pretty, and date guys. Come on—admit it now—aren't these desires deep within each of us somewhere? As we seek to find what a fellow wants and needs, we're going to find out that he wants *you!* I can just see the shocked expression forming on your face. There *is* a guy out there somewhere just for you!

God has him picked out, and is preparing him right now to be just what you want and need. Somewhere, sometime you are going to meet him. The very next place you go may be that special time and place. Exciting, isn't it? Don't be depressed if you havn't found him yet. Just think, every time you get ready to go somewhere you may be getting ready to go meet your "special" fellow. Ugh—did you think of that last night when you ran down to the market for your mom in cut-offs and T-shirt, with hair stringing down your back?

Girls go to college to educate themselves for special vocations; yet for marriage—a lifetime decision—training has been neglected. Trying to better yourself in this special way is not selfish. You owe it to yourself—and to the man you will someday marry—to reach your highest potential. The greatest aim you can have is to marry and have a loving home —to be the best wife and homemaker possible. Your benefits will be feelings of pride, accomplishment, and confidence. Your man is rewarded by bringing out the real love that he has within—giving him a new meaning in life. His need to shelter and protect will be met. He will have the incentive to do the utmost he can in the very best way he can, just for you. With the confidence of feeling more like a man, he can excel in any endeavor knowing that you are standing behind him with your support.

Smile! You Are Somebody

Boys have different tastes but the standard appeals are the same to all. We're not going to try to cut one pattern and make every girl universal. *Be Yourself!* Fakes are obvious, and guys have a peculiar way of sensing this.

"But I wish I had Karen's long, blond hair"; or, "If only I had Diane's perfect complexion." Ever found yourself wishfully making these comments? There's really no need to, because you very likely have some quality other girls long for and admire. Make the most of what you have. Bring out your hidden qualities and attractions. Emphasize the differences in your appearance and character instead of minimizing them. A big mistake I made was to select someone whom I considered to be the "ideal" and set out to be just like her. I began a full-fledged campaign to pattern myself after her talk, walk, clothes, and entire personality. How frustrated I became after a few days of consistently failing to mimic her style. Sure, I could keep up the act for a few hours pretty well, but when I'd lose concentration my true self would shine through. A feeling of failure overwhelmed me because I couldn't be what I admired in that "ideal" girl.

"How can she keep it up all the time?" I thought. But she wasn't putting on an act, as I had been doing. What I saw was the real person, not a programmed personality. When I first realized I could be myself and be happy at it, I was truly relieved. In order for others to like and accept me, I discovered I had to like and accept myself.

With this new confidence I began to be more at ease among friends, especially fellows. Try it. You have to live with yourself, so you may as well be your own best friend. If you continuously downgrade yourself to others, they'll start believing you.

One girl in our church youth department complained week after week about her "stringy hair that I can't do anything with." Upon meeting her, I had thought, "What a sweet attractive girl." After several weeks of hearing about her hair, I found myself thinking, "She certainly would look prettier with a different hairstyle." In fact, I began to even find flaws in other areas of her appearance. I had been pressured into negative thinking by the girl herself. I heard her bad points so often that I began to think she was right.

Now I'm not advocating that you broadcast your good points on billboards, or go around with your nose stuck up in the air in a conceited way. Nor am I saying that you should accept yourself as you are and not try to make constructive improvements. However, if there is something about you that is impossible to change, *Accept it* as such and make the most of it by emphasizing your positive characteristics. A girl friend I met in college has a very severe burn covering practically the entire right side of her face. Yet to know this sweet girl you would think she never gave the burn a second thought. She is a humorous, very friendly girl with a ready smile that makes you overlook her facial scarring. She accepted the burn and decided to have a radiant smile and attitude, so that people rarely even notice anything else about her.

You can change many things about yourself and your appearance. However, some things are here to stay. There is one detail about myself that I definitely wish I could make disappear, but I know I can't. I have never mentioned it to anyone, and as a result have never had it brought out in the open. I just accept it and don't emphasize it. By doing this I even forget about its existence myself!

Take a look at yourself through the eyes of a fellow. Guys *are* different, you know! And they *do* look carefully from head to toe. The eye stimulus is a male's strongest emotion. He looks at things completely differently than we girls do. Have you ever known a girl that so many guys think is really sharp-looking—one who gets all the dates? You can't figure out what they think is so great about her; you think other girls are much prettier. But there she is with the sharpest guys in the school chasing her. What is the special something that determines whether a boy asks a girl out or not? Then there are others that may think you are nice, but treat you like their sister or cousin. What's missing?

Probably the most obvious quality fellows first notice about a girl is whether or not she is different from "the guys." Opposites attract; for example: soft versus harsh, gentle versus rough, dependency versus self-reliance.

What a girl wears, how her hair is combed, and how a girl talks are details certainly noticed by men. What will attract them most, however, is not that overall outward appearance. It is the charm of radiance in a girl's face and eyes that draws his attention in an irresistible way. Sure, a boy will notice a cute girl standing on the other side of the room (all guys are girl-watchers). But the difference between a glance and a look is often determined by the look on *her* face. How appealing does a girl look when she is standing among friends gazing off into space with a dull, bored expression? Compare her with the girl who is joining in conversation, eyes sparkling with excitement and interest. Which girl would the fellows select for a date? A girl appearing dull and uninteresting never attracts any guy, no matter how beautiful she is.

Perhaps you feel that this is just not you—that you aren't the exciting, radiant person just described. It doesn't come naturally for most people. Practice smiling in front of your mirror. You'll feel like a nut at first—smiling at yourself! But when it becomes natural in the privacy of your own bedroom, you will be smiling at others naturally when in a group. Now I don't mean to pour it on so thick that others get nauseated at your sugarcoated sweetness. Your facial expressions and smile should be genuine, not overdone, so that you will be a very pleasant person to be around—and others will *want* to be around you because of your cheerful attitude.

Thinking pleasant thoughts and having a positive outlook (even on days when things go wrong) will keep your countenance cheerful. I can always tell what kind of day my girls have had by the way they walk through the doors of our church. What's on the inside shows through on the outside. Try not to be pessimistic or skeptical with life in general. Put emphasis on optimism and the brighter side of life, and you won't be able to help but be radiant. We all know people who enter a room and gloom takes over. Such negative moods are very contagious. But so is radiance! You have the power to lift others' spirits and bring sunshine into their cloudy day. There are more than enough sad, depressed people in the world. Wise was the person who said, "A bright smile does more good for the downhearted than does food for the hungry."

Girl Friend or Mother-Image?

Now that we've seen what a guy wants, let's see what he really needs. Before a fellow and girl can be romantically involved, they need to be friends. Guys want someone to whom they can talk freely and with confidence. Be a good listener. Look at him when he talks to you so that he knows that you are listening to what he is saying and nothing else. This shows him that what he says is important to you and you care. Boys need a girl who can listen to their every dream and goal without criticizing or advising. If you criticize or advise, he is reminded of his mother and no guy can get romantic with a mother-image.

One girl shared with me that she followed the advice to listen and cling to every word her boyfriend said. She found him talking on and on about many things he'd never mentioned before in their six months of dating steadily. He'd kept these things inside and never brought them up before, because she seemed so preoccupied. While he was trying to pour out his innermost feelings, she had always been busy filing her nails or thumbing through a magazine. So he quit trying. Their relationship was deeply enriched when she began practicing this listening technique.

Another girl tried this on the first date with a basically shy, quiet guy. Responding to her sincere comments as she listened he said, "I don't know why I told you all this. I've never told anyone before. It just came out."

It just "came out" because the girl had made it easy for him to talk. She showed him that he could say anything and she would not cut him down for it. A fellow needs such loyalty and trust in a girl before he can make her a special girl friend. He has to know she won't go running to her friends to tell them everything he has shared with her the night before. When this confidence is betrayed, he may clam up or find someone else in whom he can confide.

Just as we girls like to know that we look nice and pretty, a guy wants to hear admiration and praise for his accomplishments and looks. What your man wants to know most of all is that you admire him for his abilities, dreams, and ideas. If you, as his girl friend, do not supply such admiration, he will go to someone else for it. It is something he cannot give himself. He likes receiving it from any source, but most of all from that special girl. Don't wait for him to have to hint around trying to coax the praise out of you. Of all things, be most unselfish with words of admiration. Never be too busy or preoccupied to notice things about your fellow that deserve praise.

To the teenage male, praise of manly qualities is so important. He will be disappointed if you do not notice and admire his masculinity, especially his physique. Be fascinated with his large muscles, deep voice, mustache, large hands, and so forth, and *let him know it.* Take opportunity to praise his efforts in sports, mowing the lawn, or opening a tight jar lid.

Admiration of traits which are common to men and women mean little to a man. It is not nearly as important that he is kind and pleasant, as it is that he can run around the bases faster than any other guy on the team. He will appreciate any praise, but nothing will boost his ego as much as the admiration of his masculine qualities.

I have personally often seen a girl encourage her boyfriend before a ball game, urging him to go out to win "just for me."

And I've seen that boyfriend do just that. Such confidence gives guys the energy and incentive to do their best. This makes a girl feel really needed, knowing that she has the power to bring out the best in someone, doesn't it?

A fellow is very proud of his masculine traits, and likes to show them off in front of you, and anyone else who will take notice. So be sure to take notice! He cannot bear to be belittled by you and suffer humiliation. He will feel tenderness toward the girl who makes him have a wonderful sense of manliness, and be turned off by a girl who crushes his ego. In sports, guys often belittle each other to build themselves up. When he has gone through a day like this he will look to you to restore his pride.

Don't make the mistake of making fun of anything having to do with your guy's masculinity—his appearance or his accomplishments. "But," you say, "I can't find anything manly about him." Every truly feminine girl can find masculinity somewhere in every guy she meets. If you can't find anything masculine in him, chances are he won't see anything womanly in you. Once you get in the habit of being on the lookout for these qualities, you will not find any boy uninteresting. Every person has the right to be accepted just as he or she is. A fellow especially needs to know that his girl friend is not going to try to remake him into something he is not. The girl he selects for his own must be willing to accept him at face value.

Accept his ideas, accept his dreams, even his little personality quirks (and we all have those, don't we!). Don't offer little hints and suggestions for improvement. Any indication that you are not satisfied with him will drive him to another girl—someone who can accept everything about him. No guy likes the feeling of being pushed—above all, by a girl.

Every boy is going to be human and have some faults. Don't have the "Pollyanna outlook" of trying to convince yourself that he is perfect. You will be sadly disappointed. If you cannot accept a guy as he is, it may be better for you to find someone whom you can accept at face value.

Your Curb Appeal

We've seen what a guy wants and needs; next let's examine how you can attain these traits. A male is first attracted by sight, so let's start with outer appearance. When you are confident that you look your best, then you can concentrate on the other person.

Remember, a male thinks differently than we gals do. Before he can care about you, he has to first get past the visual barrier of how you look. A guy wants a girl whose physical appearance he can be proud of when he goes places; he wants to show off his date to the other onlooking guys. The outer shell you live in is what real-estate people call "curb appeal." How is *your* curb appeal? When you look sharp your countenance and attitude say, "Pick me! I'm the ideal date."

"A little fresh paint never hurt any barn door" is a wise, old farm-town saying. Most girls were not born with naturally radiant cheeks, curly eyelashes, and rosy moist lips. It's because of this that we all can stand some "fresh paint."

Using makeup appropriately can be your best appearance asset. Makeup can bring out your best features and minimize your faults. Some girls only need a little cheek blush, eye mascara, and lip gloss to achieve the fresh, natural look that guys notice.

Occasional complexion problems can be de-emphasized by a cover-up stick. Don't make the mistake of pouring on tons of liquid makeup or powder to cover these problems. Usually it only makes them more obvious and your face looks stiff and unnatural. Don't fret! You will soon be past the teen complexion-problem stage and have a glowing, blemish-free face. Many girls have these problems only during their monthly periods. During this time wash your face extra often, and keep excess oils removed with astringent. It may be wise even to carry a small bottle and cotton balls in your purse for a cleansing in between classes at school. If severe breaking-out persists, encourage your parents to invest in your seeing a dermatologist. If such a condition lingers and is untreated, it is possible that scars or pitting will be permanent.

In teaching a Christian charm course, I applied a moderate amount of makeup, touching up a girl's cheeks with a little blush, her eyes with eyeliner and mascara, and her lips with a moist lip gloss. This girl had not been accustomed to wearing any makeup at all. *What a difference!* She looked alive, whereas before she had appeared sickly and unappealing. To a second girl, I thickly brushed on eye shadow, used lots of foundation, and bright lipstick. She looked ready for a masquerade party. It was obvious which girl looked nicer. Too much makeup turns a guy off. When a girl lays her head on his shoulder, he doesn't want to have to brush the excess makeup off his sweater. Nor does he want to feel like he's dating a clown in costume.

The key to the art of using makeup is *naturalness*. Use discretion! Select tones that closely match your facial and hair coloring. What may look great on that girl friend or TV commercial may not necessarily look great on you.

Consider some points when selecting a hairstyle. The present fad may not suit the shape of your face or your personality. *Be yourself.* Select the length and style that best suit you.

Vary your hair style by adding ribbons, scarfs, and barrettes often. Such additions close to the face attract fellows by suggesting a soft, feminine effect. Keep your hair away from your face so you don't give the impression of a rag mop or shaggy dog.

Is it true that blonds have more fun? Every girl has the temptation to change her hair color in order to make herself more exciting. A tint or rinse can often enhance natural beauty, but avoid drastically changing your hair color. Many girls regret the change afterward and have to suffer through the long growing-out process of the roots. When others see that you have so little confidence in yourself that you even have to change your hair color, they lose respect for you. Subconciously they figure you will try to cover up other important matters. You will feel cheapened and fake knowing the drastic change is not really you. Again I stress naturalness, for this attracts more than false beauty.

Most of us don't have the money to get an entire new wardrobe every time the styles change, so make what you do buy count. Don't buy on the spur of the moment or just because it's on sale. Make sure the fit, style, and color is just what you want.

Wear styles that contrast to men's apparel and accent femininity. When you wear pants, soften the effect by choosing a feminine color and accessories. Avoid severely tailored styles or other suggestions of masculinity. Too often girls only wear pants or jeans and are never seen in dresses. Take advantage of that fact that dresses are appealing to guys, mainly because they do not wear them! Dresses of soft cottons, designs, floral prints, and polka dots are always attractive. Avoid those that are gaudy and lack good taste. Some girls look overdressed in loud colors and dominating designs. Extreme feminine styles include ruffles, puffs, and gathers. Combine these with your styles when in fashion.

The material that your outfit is made of can set off the soft look also. Color is extremely important. Brown, black, and navy, unless set off by a brighter color can be very unappealing. A stylish outfit that all your girl friends envy may not necessarily bring admiration from the fellows. What initially attracts their attention is softness, airiness, and delicacy. I've always noticed these qualities in the clothing my husband selects for me. Some of my outfits that are not the most stylish are the ones that bring the most compliments, because of how feminine they make me look and feel. The greater the contrast to masculinity, the more striking the effect. Regardless of what the unisex advocates say, men still like to go out with someone who looks like a *girl—not a guy!*

I've heard and read of many examples to support this truth. One girl is said to have walked down a street and into the same store twice. The first time she had on a stylish brown outfit with shoes and purse to match. She walked into the store attracting no attention whatsoever. A little later the same girl walked along the crowded street into the same store in a colorful, feminine dress with her hair loosely hanging down her back and tied with a pink ribbon. She was entertained and surprised to experience the difference made by the change of outfits. She noticed the glances from the young men who passed her along the way. A man at the store even offered her a job as cashier. The second outfit consisted of color and style contrary to what men would wear themselves. This outfit emphasized the fact that she was a girl; it was the essence of femininity. Every guy is interested in girls who give such an impression in their outward appearance.

Your wardrobe should include a variety of separates that can be mixed and matched to form new outfits. Have styles for different occasions from sporty to formal. Keep the element of surprise alive in your dress. Maybe one day dress in a sophisticated manner and the next day your outfit can be little-girlie.

Here is some wise advise I received one time: *A guy can stand just about anything except boredom.* Don't let your fellow get bored with your way of dressing. You can be exciting by the variety in your outfits. He will never know how to expect you dressed next, and the change will keep him anxious to see you.

Your outfit should obviously speak for itself. It should say,

"Today I am soft, little-girlie"; or, "Today I am casual and sporty." Such variations do not have to be expensive if you start with the basic items and go from there to add and accent.

Sewing your own apparel brings pride and originality. Your fellow will be proud to hear you say, "I made it myself." Knowing how to sew also comes in handy when clothes start to show their wear. Nothing looks worse than a beautiful dress with a hem hanging down or a seam bursting out. Fix places that need mending before hanging the garments up. This assures that the outfit will be ready to wear the next time you hurriedly select it. Don't get in the habit of pinning either; this always looks ungroomed. An overall neat appearance is important to turn his eye. Guys are not inclined to mend tears and sew on buttons, but they expect tidiness of their girls. Strive to appear your best every minute of the day —yes—under all circumstances.

Many girls are encouraged, even by their mothers, to look, act, and dress sexy. In spite of the emphasis placed on the Sex Symbol today, guys still respect the girl who does not expose herself publicly. Sure, dressing sexy with plunging necklines and miniskirts will turn the men's eyes, but that kind of cheap attraction and attention is not a result of respect, nor does it produce respect. Girls who act and dress immodestly may get a lot of dates, but when the guys look for someone whom they can be proud of, they do not go for these girls. A boy wants a girl who is his very own, his "special girl," not someone every other fellow feasted his eyes on.

I read of a group of high-school boys who made this report about girls they had observed:

> We have been girl-watching for the past four weeks. Much of what we have seen has displeased,

disgusted, and disappointed us. We are tired of constantly being forced to look at girls' underwear. Boys do not like the carelessness girls display when sitting or stooping. This is no thrill—just obnoxious.

We find girls draped in boys' clothing unattractive and unfeminine. Wear your own clothes and let us wear ours.

We take a dim view of girls using profane and obscene language in their conversation. Clean up your mouths or keep quiet.

We are concerned about the large number of girls whose general behavior is becoming increasingly unfeminine and boylike. Girls who greet us by pushing us, hitting us, or pounding us on the back leave us cold. Try just saying hello.

Clear enough, gals? Harshly spoken and to the point—right? Did you find yourself falling into any of the mentioned categories? It may seem that the sexy route is the way to follow as far as dress and actions are concerned. But it turns a guy off—anyone worth having, that is!

Dressing in an outfit that exposes much of your bust and legs leaves nothing to the imagination. When you sit next to a date in a car, he certainly won't be thinking about that algebra test he has tomorrow. The girl sets the mood on a date. Through your conversation and actions you are telling a boy, "Come on, I'm yours"; or, "Hands off!" When a suggestive signal reaches him, no guy can help himself. He *will* react! When you snuggle up close, the softness and warmth of your body is too tempting not to touch. And girls, we're human too! You say, "I will stop before we go too far. I can control my emotions." I've heard that statement far too often. Many unwed mothers made the same claim before they found out too late.

Me, Myself, and I!

I always tell my students in TOTAL GIRL classes that if any of them should get herself in trouble, I will be there to help in any way I can. But, I add, "Don't tell me it wasn't your fault." It's up to you, girls, not to let yourselves be placed in the position where something could too easily happen. And it happens so fast! I've heard those words time and again, "It was over before I knew what was happening." If you stay away from places where a date could too easily take advantage of you (drive-ins, apartments, parked cars), then you won't be ashamed to face yourself the next morning. And morning *does* come!

Snack-Snitchers

It will make no difference what kind of outfit you are wearing if what's inside of the outfit isn't appealing. Don't get into the habit of sneaking snacks now, or later it will show! Not all of us have Raquel Welch figures, but that doesn't mean we can't stop trying!

Along with watching what you eat, the ideal figure requires exercising. This is not just for the excessively overweight girls either. Exercising really helps tone muscles and gives an overall healthy appearance. If weight is one adjustment you need to make in your appearance—*Start Now!* Perhaps even go to a doctor for the best plan. There will be no easier time than now to begin; in fact each year the pounds get harder to lose. You'll look better, feel better, and do better!

Using all these attention-getting pointers you will catch your fellow's attention with your attractive appearance. Now don't ruin his favorable impressions by your actions, your walk, voice, eyes, and movements.

A girl's walk needs to be light and airy—not the quick, heavy gait of a man. I'm not suggesting that girls everywhere go around with books supported on top of their heads either. Yet a good walk requires good posture by properly holding the head and shoulders. The girl who drags into a room slouching, slumping, and sliding her feet along will not make a favorable impression. She will appear depressed, dull, and all fizzled out. Then there's the girl who barges into a room as though she has been shot from a cannon. She practically skips from person to person nervously shouting and laughing at the top of her lungs. When she exits, everyone is exhausted from watching this tornado blow through. Try to strike a happy medium in contrast to these two girls. Most of all, avoid the swaying of your shoulders and arms and the long strides that reflect the walk of a man.

Gentleness in the way you use your hands is a feminine way of expressing yourself. Overfirmness when shaking hands or holding hands is to be avoided. Your hands are noticed more than you may be aware of, so strive to acquire gentle motions. This is especially important when waving to someone, gesturing in conversation, and when eating. Never use stiff, jerky movements or pound on a table when speaking. And by all means don't go around slapping boys on the back! This would remind them of a fellow-football player instead of a possible date. Gentle maneuvers charm men because they accentuate the differences between them and yourself, rather than similarities.

Femininity has been defined as "a gentle, tender quality." Speaking or laughing loudly and firmly spoils the feminine effect, no matter how dainty a girl's appearance may be. I don't mean that girls should speak in a whisper or timidly, for this shows a lack of self-assurance. No fellow likes to carry on a conversation with a monotonous singsong voice either. This makes a girl seem dull and uninteresting. Practice speaking to yourself, or even read aloud to gain expression and enthusiasm in your voice. Endeavor to eliminate monotony. When you are in conversation you will find the emotion coming out naturally and automatically.

Time to Spare

Feeling swamped under with improvements that need to be made? I know the feeling. You feel like you'll never have time to date—even if you do get asked out—because of all the assignments you need to be working on. You need a plan. You need the plan that Ivy Lee, a management consultant, devised. He received twenty-five thousand dollars for suggesting it to the president of his company!

The Twenty-five-Thousand-Dollar Plan

1. Every night write down the important things you need to get accomplished the next day.
2. Number them in order as to importance. (Clean room, housework, wash hair, etc.)
3. Next day, finish as much on your plan as is possible. Do the hardest tasks first.
4. When interruptions come, accept them, then go right on trying to finish each item.

This plan of organization will enable you to go out when that special boy asks you unexpectedly. You will be calm and unrushed, because you will have had your important jobs completed. Won't Mom be thrilled when you have accomplished much more than ever before—and without her even yelling at you repeatedly! With this new feeling of accomplishment, you will have pampering time for yourself. You will be able to keep your nails groomed, give yourself facial masks, brush your hair to a healthy glow, and even soak in a bubble bath. Most of all your attitude will turn your work into fun. I actually get a thrill every day as I get to check off the points on my list as I finish my tasks. I challenge myself to complete my whole list. Try The Twenty-five-Thousand-Dollar Plan for a week. See if your attitude doesn't change. *And* notice the remaining time allowed to devote to yourself!

Homework 1

1. Practice **The Twenty-Five-Thousand-Dollar Plan** every day for a week.

2. Make one noticeable change for the better in your outer appearance.

3. Practice smiling at yourself in front of your mirror every morning. Determine to be a more pleasant-looking and-speaking person.

4. Try to give five sincere compliments each day. You'll feel much better and so will those around you.

2

Securing His Attention

The first time a fellow notices you will always stick in his mind. Make it count! My husband, Rob, loves to recall the first time he caught sight of me (I kind of enjoy hearing it over and over again, too). Rob dramatizes the scene as he tells how I was standing in the long freshmen registration line the first day of college. Being an "experienced junior," Rob, with some colleagues, was scouting out the freshmen-dating possibilities. There I was—I must have really stood out—not because of my looks but for my stupidity. With my hands full of papers, books, and cards, I didn't know which end was up. I was so lost, and felt so insecure, especially since I did not know a soul. Rob gloats as he recalls how he pointed that blond out to his friends saying, "I'm going to date her!" Sure enough, he did and we're still dating as man and wife. Whenever you leave your house, remember that you may be making your first impression on someone important. Like me, you may not even be aware that you are being observed.

Right Place, Right Time

Boys probably have not been flocking to you, or knocking down your front door to meet you. It just doesn't work that way. A stay-at-home never gets dates. Involve yourself in school activities, church and social clubs. Take notice of girl friends who can introduce you to male friends or even older brothers.

When you get to an activity make sure you take part and don't just sit on the sidelines. Wallflowers just don't convey much excitement. Stand out in an attractive manner in contrast with the other girls by your feminine actions. If a group of girls you are with is shouting loudly, you can contrast this by being gentle and demure. Such actions will be favorably noticed by fellows. Boys will type you along with the other girls, if you associate with their unattractive ways. Don't be associated with friends who will detract from your character by their poor actions.

A proper and effective method of attracting a boy's attention is calling upon him for assistance. Chances are, if you try a task alone, he will come to your aid before you have to ask. Denise successfully used this technique one afternoon as our church youth group was decorating for a banquet. Being rather short, it was a difficult task for her to hang crepe-paper streamers from the ceiling, even standing on a chair. Observing her difficulty, Ken lowered her from the chair and insisted on hanging the streamers himself. I watched as they had an enjoyable conversation getting to know each other while Denise handed Ken the streamers to hang. As a result, Ken escorted Denise to that very banquet.

A guy always wants everything to be *his* own preconceived idea. Never be too obvious or aggressive when you are introduced to a boy, or when gaining his attention. If he feels that you had it in the back of your mind that someday you would date, it will be like *you* are asking *him* out. He would feel as though he had no say in the matter. This steals his masculinity and robs him of his self-respect.

Do not limit your friendships to people of your own age. Older folks have sons and nephews. Children have uncles and older brothers. That child whom you baby-sit may have a relative who is excellent dating material. Every man, woman, and child you meet may have a relative or friend you might be interested in meeting. By limiting your acquaintances, you narrow your dating possibilities.

A very effective means of meeting new people is giving a party yourself. Invite your friends and encourage them to bring along a new friend or two of their own. You can meet many fellows at social affairs because introductions are the proper procedure when unknown folks enter. You, as the hostess, will get to know everyone present and be in the spotlight for boys to talk with more easily.

How ideal a date you may be makes no difference unless boys are aware of you—and your appearance and personality suggest that you'll be fun to take out. Just as a manufacturer advertises his product so that people will buy it, you must make guys aware that you exist before they can ask you out. You must, however, call attention to yourself in a feminine manner, not in a bold aggressive way. This would backfire by cheapening your image in his eyes. Your appearance, the places you go, and the first conversation you have will determine whether or not you are a desirable date.

Winning His Initial Interest

Those first flirtations are exciting, scary, and fun! You just know he's noticed you, but now what? Oh, no! Here he comes across the room. Is he coming your way? Crumb! He's gone to the food table. But wait a minute! He's picked up two sandwiches. Well, maybe he eats a lot. No, he's walking in this direction. Oh, no! Do you look at him shyly? No—he may think you are too forward. Do you look the other way? No—he may think that you couldn't care less if he came over to talk to you. He's standing right in front of you. Your knees tremble, and you're very glad he suggests sitting down. Now what? You can't sit there forever munching on the sandwich. What do you say?

Arouse his interest by remarking on something he did with a compliment. If he plays football, admire his strong throwing ability. If he has just received an A on a test, remark about how hard he must have studied. If you have just been introduced to this eligible young man, ask him a question. This will get the conversation going with him taking part. He will feel superior and manly when you present him with the chance to explain something to you. As he speaks, really listen to him by looking right at him, commenting occasionally. He will feel as if you are really interested in him as a person, and feel important to you right at the start of your relationship.

Suggest action for the two of you—something you can do together. Maybe you can join in a game being played by the group, or get something from the refreshment table. Doing something together establishes you both as a couple.

Perhaps you could even assist your fellow in a job that he is doing. If a group is working on a project, try to join in his area of work. By working together he will think, "I just can't do this again without her." Cheer just for him at the game, and he will play just to gain your attention and approval. Then the next time he undertakes this task that you've assisted with, he will seek you out and want you there again.

The First Big Date

You smile at yourself as you excitedly put the phone back on the receiver, then dash into the kitchen to relate the wonderful news! "He finally asked me out," you exclaim, going further into detail about this upcoming date.

One word of caution—don't be too eager when the guy of your dreams does finally make the move. Accept the date with pleasure, but don't make it sound like you have been sitting on top of the telephone waiting for it to ring. Be friendly with other boys at school while you are being friendly with him. This way, he will never quite know if you really like only him. Keep him guessing at first—this is intriguing to a fellow. Don't accept a lot of dates right at the start, and don't appear overanxious to get serious. Arrange to have "other plans." Show an interest in hobbies, your job, and other activities. This will relieve him of thinking you are bored with life and possibly husband-hunting.

Before the first date you may be uneasy about conversation topics, especially if you have just met him. It never hurts actually to list on paper hints for topics to bring up. Arouse his interest in you by winning his confidence through conversation. Remember—the best conversationalists are the best listeners! Take mental notes of manly points about him that you can admire. As he talks, show understanding and appreciation of what he relates to you. Be interested in the topics he brings up and share common interests. Selfishness has no place in dating. Delight in his sports, ambitions, and aspirations. Even try to laugh at his jokes—no matter how corny they may be or how many times you've heard them!

Never, *never* be late for a date, especially a first date. When you are late, he doesn't have time to admire how nice you look, meet your parents properly, or drive sensibly. Dating cannot be rushed without the consequence of creating pressures on the couple and placing a tension in the atmosphere. Be on time in order to start the evening in a calm, unrushed manner. You will *both* be more at ease and will be able to be yourselves. A guy wants to be able to relax with a girl and not have to hurry through the evening feeling like he's in a fast motion picture.

When fellows are asked what quality they would most like their date to have, the majority answer with one word. Not *pretty,* but *fun.* Dull, uninteresting girls rarely get asked for a second date. Would you ask yourself out? Are you fun enough to create the desire for future dates? Even the liveliest party can be dull for a boy, if his date makes dull conversation and likes to sit on the sidelines. Strive to be fun and enthusiastic without being aggressive.

Aggressiveness deprives a fellow of his masculinity. Let him make the moves whether it involves where you go or the good-night kiss. When he asks your opinion, offer it, but don't insist on getting your way. Submission is *not* letting a boy tramp on you like a floor mat. You'll find that when you submit to your dates suggestions and ideas, later he'll want to do anything to please you. He will ask your ideas about even the important matters.

Handing out kisses and cuddling up close to boys on dates makes you appear aggressive and eager. This makes a fellow feel like you are just using him to satisfy your female desires. Dating is a period of transition, not a time of sampling physical curiosities. There should be a spiritual relationship in dating wherein each partner can better serve the Lord having shared His blessings together. This will leave the boy with a respectful feeling toward you rather than a cheap impression.

During the period when affections for each other are growing rapidly, it is easy for a girl and guy to let emotions take hold. Emotions were meant to accompany love, not come before it. Letting emotions take control will confuse you both and make the relationship progress too rapidly. Remember, you will always do more with a fellow on the next date than you did on the last. It is like taking up where you left off, so start out slow. Your guy will wonder, "Has she given out to every guy like this?" By holding on to your expressions and affections, you will establish respect in his eyes.

Giving in to emotions leads to passion and lust, especially on the part of a guy. You, as a girl, set the mood on a date.

Your actions will either be saying, "I'm yours"; or "Hands off!" The signals are obvious and he will read them fast. When you "turn on" a guy by letting him touch and fondle your body, he becomes passionate both physically and emotionally. All systems are go and he won't be easily turned off.

Everybody's Not Doing It!

"But," you claim, "abstaining from sex is so old-fashioned. There's the new morality now—free love, sexual freedom." Even if we don't consider the eventual consequences, God commands us to save the sexual relationship for marriage. This God-ordained communion between man and woman is sacred. Fornication is still a sin in God's eyes, regardless of what man has allowed to be accepted in society. Giving sex before marriage cheapens a fellow's opinion of you. You will be no challenge to him. The unattainable girl presents a challenge to a guy. He will want to date you again and again, instead of dropping you after "getting what you had to give."

"But, everybody's doing it." That is a very invalid assumption. Of the unmarried girls in the United States, ages fifteen to nineteen, only 28 percent have ever actually had sexual intercourse, according to an article in *Seventeen* magazine (June, 1974). The girls who have indulged in premarital sex are usually seeking self-confidence or popularity. A pretty high-school junior related to me, "I went all the way on my dates because all my friends said that's just what you were supposed to do. Seems like they aren't even my friends any more." Using sex as a means to gain popularity will always backfire.

"To keep my boyfriend I had to go to bed with him. He said he would find someone else who would if I didn't." My advice to that girl was, "Let him!" Many girls yield because they are afraid of losing a guy by saying no to him. The opposite is true. Some girls tell me that they "hurt his feelings by not giving in to him." But, consider the way he's hurting your feelings! More often than not, once a fellow has gotten what he feels he can from a girl, he will go on to the next girl who will offer him what he wants. Many girls are heartbroken when they find out they've just been used and sweet-talked into giving in.

Consider the consequences of a sexual relationship between you and a fellow. Losing your virginity is losing your most precious possession. Someday you will want to give it to that one and only special man. If you've already lost this possession in an unmeaningful relationship, you will not have it to offer when it counts. Consider the possibility of pregnancy. Are you ready to face that responsibility? And more often than not—alone. Can you handle the guilt? Do not base your desires on false premises. Just because a guy says he wants you for a bed partner, you can't be assured he desires you for a marriage partner. Many girls make the mistake of believing that if they give themselves away in sex, they will hold their fellow's interest and eventually win a mate.

Biblical Restraint

You *can* care for someone and he for you without having sex. Sexual surrender is not the secret to winning a man. It is worth waiting for, even if it does mean losing a date or two right now. Knowing you'll have gratitude and respect from your "Mr. Right" in the future makes it a little easier to abstain right now. Keep that thought as a high goal ever present in your mind. If it is still hard to say no—especially if you have been accustomed to giving in—you may want to follow one of my girls' examples. Cindy and Dave had dated seriously for over a year. They were getting deeply involved sexually, and realized they had to come to a halt or suffer heartbreaking consequences. Determined to restrain their feelings from getting too carried away, they kept a Bible placed on the car seat between them on every date for a month. If it takes something that drastic—apply it! The restraint of God's Word certainly worked for Cindy and Dave.

Love is climaxed for marriage partners in a beautiful sexual union. God has planned it that way. Without true love and commitment, sex cannot have its full beauty. To the contrary, it would have very little meaning.

First John 4:18 states: ". . . perfect love casteth out fear . . . ." A wife can give herself to her partner because she trusts him, and there is no fear in their relationship. It is not a purely physical attraction that will lose hold after a while. God intends for men and women to delight in the physical aspect of their marital union. This is beauty, this is trust, this is love.

> And now abideth faith, hope, and [love], these three; but the greatest of these is [love].
>
> 1 Corinthians 13:13

Homework 2

1. List common-interest conversation topics on paper, so you will be prepared when the time comes.

2. Buy something new for your wardrobe. Make it something feminine in color and style.

3. Don't be a stay-at-home. Attend as many school and church functions as your time will allow.

4. Set one specific goal for yourself. Determine to accomplish this goal within one week.

> I have just a minute,
> Only sixty seconds in it,
> Forced upon me—
> Can't refuse it—
> Didn't choose it—
> But it's up to me to use it.
> I must suffer if I lose it,
> Give account if I abuse it,
> Just a tiny little minute,
> But eternity is in it.
>
> **AUTHOR UNKNOWN**

3

Creative Dating

Nothing encourages a guy to look for other "fish in the sea" as much as a boring dating partner. Some girls seem very attractive and interesting upon a first meeting or within the company of a group. But when they get alone with a fellow on a date, he may as well be sitting next to a marble statue. These are the girls who rarely get asked out the second or third time. They have no topics of conversation to discuss, and couldn't care less what their date is interested in or likes to do. They just want to go to the same places every Friday night or go where the gang happens to be hanging out. This type of a date will not have her door beaten down by prospects of future daters. Believe me, word travels fast among boys. There are two things they love to discuss —how great their date was, or how rotten their whole evening went. Guys don't necessarily have the idea that they will find out for themselves either. They simply take the experienced fellow's word and leave it at that.

Many girls provide good dating material during the initial few months of dating. However, after dating steadily for any length of time, it becomes easy to take a boy for granted. Dates become routine meetings instead of fun, exciting experiences. It's no wonder a fellow wants to get out of this type of relationship. He feels that some other girl could provide him with the excitement and variation he desires. But, so as to not hurt his girl friend, many guys hang on.

Dates get stale as a result of this lack of imagination, and oftentimes arguments become frequent pastimes. It's not hard to see how this situation easily develops. The same ol' car, same ol' person, and the same ol' places will naturally get boring after a while. It is up to *you* to be creative in suggesting new places to go, things to see, and activities to do.

The whole blame is not placed on the girl partner, but usually she will have to be the one to make the first move. After that, you'll find your boyfriend following your example in becoming more imaginative too. It is often really difficult for some boys to think of anything to do on a date other than attend school functions or ball games. When he sees how much fun your various suggestions can be, your date will try to come up with some new ones of his own.

Let's Celebrate!

Lack of imagination in dating is the reason many couples end up at their private parking places, getting tempted, and carried away. Most girls use the excuse that "there just isn't anything else to do" to justify "making out" all evening. Sure, it may take a little creativity and perhaps even expense on the girl's part, but the fun rewards received in doing so are well worth it. Plus, you will both be relieved from the guilt feelings that follow an evening of necking and parking.

When you begin to invent new dating ideas and plan special fun times, many rewards will accompany your efforts. Your guy will see that you really want to be with him enough to go to this extra time in planning. The message will come through loud and clear that "this is just for him." He will appreciate you and your relationship so much more by seeing that he means this much to you. You will become a lively, creative person to him—someone who can think on her own and is fun to be with. He will be anxiously awaiting each date because he knows you will have some great new idea up your sleeve.

Don't always go to the same pizza parlor or hamburger drive-in after the games. Suggest trying new places with various types of foods and atmosphere. Enjoy the outdoors by going on hikes, bicycle rides and picnics. Have special candlelight dinners for your boyfriend to celebrate birthdays and other holidays. It's even fun to make up your own special holidays, just for the two of you to celebrate together.

One idea of an original holiday was tried by Carol, a girl attending the TOTAL GIRL classes. She declared a "Happy Day" celebration and created a very enjoyable day for herself and her steady. Carol pasted smiley faces all over her boyfriend's car and she and Bob wore matching smiley-faced T-shirts that evening on their date. All day long when they passed at school, they were to greet one another with a big smile. They each had a ball! Carol reported that it was the funniest, happiest day of their entire year of dating.

Another girl planned an exotic luau with all the Hawaiian works! She met her boyfriend at the door with a kiss, and placed a lei around his neck. Several other couples were also invited to share in the festivities for an unusual date.

You may even mention silly, impossible date ideas to him. The next time he asks you what you would like to do on Friday night answer, "I'd love to climb to the top of the highest mountain in the world and slide all the way down." He'll love to imagine you both sliding down that mountain, even though it is impossible.

My husband, Rob, is as fun-loving as husbands come. All through our marriage we have had our weekly "date night." He calls me from work and asks me out, then picks me up —just like when we were single. One day I remarked how beautiful the fall leaves were as they changed color and fell to the ground. I remember saying how much fun it would be to bunch up big piles of leaves and run and jump in them. You guessed it! That night we had so much fun running and jumping in piles of leaves!

Michelle and Ken were really in a dating rut. Most of their dates were spent at the high-school football games. Ken was an avid sports fan, so his eyes were glued to the game, letting nothing distract him. Meanwhile, Michelle tried to seem interested, but kept her attention mostly on the cheerleaders as she munched on her popcorn. After the games, the car almost automatically drove to a secluded park just outside of town. Michelle almost broke up with Ken because of this date routine, but she really liked him a lot. She realized it was up to her to change the scene, so she got to work! She suggested different places to go after the games with their friends. She even had a "fifth-quarter" party at her house with a group of friends from school. Ken showed interest and a lot of appreciation. He began planning various types of dates and not just ball games. When Ken saw that Michelle was concerned about their relationship, he also took action.

Sue told one TOTAL GIRL Class of a surprise she presented Gary, her steady. They had planned a dinner date at a particular restaurant where a good friend of Sue's was a waitress. With her cooperation, Gary received a little surprise gift with each course of the meal. The following week Gary did a little gift-giving in the same manner. Their church youth group met at a nearby pizza parlor after the evening services. When Sue stuck her straw in her coke, she found the cup empty. Wondering why, she turned the cup upside down. Out fell a beautiful diamond engagement ring. For Sue, it certainly paid off to show a little creativity!

Filling His Cup

The main reason many marriages get stale after the first honeymoon year is because couples discontinue the fun dates. They get so wrapped up in life's daily hum-drum activities, that they forget to put in a little spice. Even in marriage, couples need to keep a special time set aside where the husband and wife can do something just by themselves.

A mother needs to forget about the children and her housework chores by directing her complete attention to her husband at least one evening a week. She should fix herself all up pretty and special just for the guy who is still Number One in her life. Without these special efforts, her husband will feel like a household fixture instead of the King of his Castle.

Many wives feel like a maid in their home and not the Queen. The husband needs to drop all work and puts business problems aside, and concentrate solely on his wife as a date for an evening at least once a week. She then no longer feels that she has lost her beauty and charm.

If you can get into the habit of making your date life fun, then your marriage will not lose its spice. Determine to be a fun dating partner—whether you are going steady or just dating around. The rewards will be yours as you reap even more fun than you sow.

Many guys are just like an empty cup that has run dry emotionally. What they need to be filled with is admiration and appreciation. All the way to the very top! Your boyfriend wants approval from friends, parents, and his coach—but most of all from *you*. You are the one he needs to make him feel special. He could be dating any other girl in school, but he picked *you* because he thought you were the most wonderful of them all. No matter how many sports or academic honors a boy receives, your admiration means more. Without it, his motivation is lost.

Start today! Determine to fill his well to the very top! He may need admiration so badly that his cup is bone-dry. Admire him as he talks to you. Look him right in the eye and express interest with short replies. Don't be preoccupied as he speaks. This shows unconcern, and eventually he will stop talking completely. Listening attentively shows that you care and what he says is important.

Above all, don't interrupt as your fellow is speaking. Maybe you couldn't care less who won yesterday's football game, but your attention in listening shows effort in being interested. Indifference shows a guy that you are selfish, and do not care to share his interests. This will turn him off fast.

Before a fellow can admire and compliment you the way you need, his own cup must be full. He must be filled to the brim before he can pour out any overflow. When his cup is running over, guess who receives this overflow? The one who has filled the cup—you!

Compliment and admire not only his physical characteristics, but also his ideals and aspirations. Tact is that special ability to describe others as they see themselves. Your boyfriend sees himself as an intellect and a sportsman with a fantastic build. He wants you to see him this way, too. The only way he'll know that you do is for you to tell him—often. This assurance of your feelings toward your fellow gives him confidence to strive harder to be even better for you. It is actually a privilege for you to assure him that he is as special to you as he had hoped.

Crown Him King

One of the most common complaints I get from girls is "my boyfriend treats me more like one of his buddies than his Queen." Probably the reason you aren't being treated like his Queen is because he isn't being made to feel like your King! This is so important to a man. How he sees his own image reflected in your eyes is essential before he can reflect the feelings back to you. It must be crystal clear in his mind that he is your hero. If he feels that he constantly has to be competing for that role, he will have no time to assure you of what you mean to him.

Psychiatrists tell us that a man's most basic needs are admiration and approval. Women need to be loved; men crave being admired. This contrast between the needs of men and women must be remembered in fulfilling the complete role of his girl friend.

Concentrate so much on his good points and his faults will somehow disappear. Don't take his good looks and manliness for granted. Try looking at him through another girl's eyes. This will bring him into focus. Give your guy several good sincere compliments a day, and watch him blossom right before your eyes. I am not advocating that you lie to give him a superficial ego boost. He will see through insincere flattery. Recall in your mind the points that first attracted you to your fellow and emphasize these to him.

Sounds to you like all we're here for is to support the male ego? Now don't get all high and mighty, and go off on a Women's Lib tangent! God made us gals with a giving, sharing, loving nature. We are to use it on our men! The Bible teaches married women actually to "reverence" their husbands. (*Read* Ephesians 5:33.) According to the dictionary, reverence means "to respect, honor, esteem, adore, praise, enjoy, and admire." Yes, this is how we are to treat our men! In actions as well as attitude and in every word.

If you can condition yourself in the practice of admiration throughout the dating period, God's command to reverence your husband will come naturally in marriage. This is what dating is all about anyway, girls. Sure, dating is fun, enjoyable, and makes you proud to be chosen by someone special. But even more than all this, dating provides a transitional period for you and some special fellow. The transitions include going from single individuality to a union which forms a couple. Throughout the dating period, both partners learn to place the other one's needs and desires above their own. Selfishness vanishes as the urge to please and serve your partner develops. Oftentimes a couple will jump prematurely into a marriage bond before this transitional period has really had time to reach its peak. Be careful of this. These marriages are commonly the ones that dissolve quickly. The strain of adjustments that should have been completed through dating are too great while living under the same roof.

This does not mean that a set time of dating can be established. Every couple will have to determine this for themselves. Circumstances such as education, family responsibilities, emotional stability, and financial security must all be considered. If he's worth loving, he's worth waiting for and vice versa.

Submission is emphasized in biblical teachings. This doesn't mean we girls are to be doormats for our guy to wipe his feet on! Far from that! But, we need to let our guys make the final decisions as to date plans concerning where to go or whom to double with, and so on. When he asks your opinion offer it, but with the assurance that you will stand by his final plan. Learning submission early in a relationship will prevent many hardships and disagreements of the roles in marriage.

God planned for a woman to be under her husband's rule. Ephesians 5:22 tells women to submit to their husbands' leadership the same way we are to submit even unto the Lord. Marriage is not 50–50, but rather giving 100 percent from each partner. God ordained marriage and set the ground rules. When these rules are applied, then *and only then* will a marriage be successful.

God's Word does not claim that women are inferior to men, as some women libbers state. God wants us to understand, however, that while men and women are equal in status, we are very different in our functions. This does not insinuate that the woman's role is unimportant or that she is to be a slave. A true woman simply realizes that a relationship needs a leader and a follower. Our female role entails various functions that men simply don't meet the qualifications to fill. The husband certainly cannot carry a baby in pregnancy and give birth at the end of nine months. Similarly, our female bodies and emotions were not intended to handle hard physical labor duties. Whereas, a man is built with the structure and strength to handle such a job.

When a woman keeps these roles in the right perspective, her man rewards her greatly. A guy appreciates a girl who sincerely wants to obey the Lord's commands in letting the male be the leader. Your man will then grant your desires just as a King who grants his Queen's every wish.

Let him know that you believe in him and trust his decisions. Don't just agree for the sake of giving in to save arguing. Tolerance is not acceptance. Don't advise by saying, "I would have . . ."; or, "Well, I think. . . ." You will sound like a second mother and no guy can be romantic with his second mother.

It is only when a woman surrenders to her man, worships him, and serves him, that she really becomes beautiful to him. She becomes his glory, his jewel, his Queen.

Mend His Wounds

There are going to be times when the whole world falls out from under your boyfriend, and he will really need your compassionate, listening ear. He will need to confide in you, tell you his deepest feelings, and let you mend his fallen ego. Be there without criticism, rejection, or advice; just be there. It can mean more to him than anything else you do.

Don't you have a special friend who is always there, ready to listen whenever you need to pour your heart out? I do. I can call her or go over to her home anytime and feel free to unload my heart to her. She wouldn't put me down; she wouldn't laugh at me. I'm free to be myself because I know she'll listen and understand.

Can we do less for our guys? Be there when he needs you! If he knows you will be, somehow life's trials will seem a little less severe. When your boyfriend's coach gives him an embarrassing, deflating lecture on how badly he played at practice—he must feel assured as he leaves the ball field that he can receive comfort simply by dialing your phone number. Without this assurance, your guy will turn to the nearest person to meet his tattered needs. And that just might be a cute, sympathetic blond! I'd sure hate to loose a fantastic fellow because I failed to provide the necessary encouragement and admiration.

No two partners in a marriage situation can always be on top of the world. There are many instances throughout life's daily routines that cause us to falter into depression. This is when two heads are better than one! The other partner can refresh and mend his mate's emotions quickly as he senses the trouble.

My two small children along with household and church responsibilities combine together in making a very hectic schedule that is sometimes humanly impossible to handle. By the time my husband, Rob, arrives home from work, some days all I can manage to do is open the door for him and say a meager *hello*. His understanding nature is just the shot in the arm that I need. By the time he has helped me feed the children and clean up after dinner, I am emotionally refreshed. Rob's willingness to encourage and assist me during the rough times enables us to then have a very enjoyable evening together.

One time I heard the importance of encouragement in a relationship illustrated by a woman like this: She explained that she or her husband would first question the other to see if they'd had a hard day. The one who was really down low could know that he would receive help from his mate. So well had they mastered these situations, that one day her husband came home and asked, "Honey, are you real tired today?" "No, not really," she replied. "Good," he answered. "Then I shall be." He knew, without a shadow of doubt, that his supporting wife would come to the rescue, but he wanted to see if she first needed his assistance.

Putting the other person first is the key. Before your boyfriend will come to you during trials, he must know you'll be there to help him. If you are constantly preoccupied only with your selfish concerns, he will not feel that talking over a problem would do any good. He will just figure that you are too wrapped up in your petty worries. Assure your guy often of your availability to listen and comfort. Sometimes he won't even need to hear a word. Your being there and lending a sympathetic ear may be enough therapy to see him through.

Yes, Let's!

Have you ever really dampened your boyfriend's suggestions by responding, "Yes, but. . . ." What a way to put him down! It doesn't matter how good your excuse was, it still has the same effect. He feels that his leadership has been challenged; he couldn't lead you and that discourages him.

The next time he makes a suggestion, respond with an enthusiastic, "Yes, let's." Whether it's deciding on a place to go or what to eat, try agreeing instead of supplying a counter idea. While he's telling you his plan, decide to accept his idea graciously. If his suggestion doesn't appeal to you, use self-control and don't disagree.

How many times have you answered to his suggestions, "What a dumb idea"; or "But I don't feel like doing that"? If you really dislike what he suggests or disagree about some plan, then simply tell him your preference. *But* let *him* make the final decision. And don't sulk the whole evening if he goes ahead with his idea instead of giving in to yours. He will be so grateful that you have given him the freedom of choice that he won't act foolishly.

Forgive and Forget

I figured that when I found my "one and only" that life would be a bed of roses forever. I soon found out that Cinderella and her Prince don't always live happily every moment of every day. There are times of misunderstanding and quarreling. These moments don't pop up only after you have been married a year either. They come even during the dating period.

Most arguments between dating couples stem from selfishness—each partner wanting his own way. This is where maturity has a lot to do with dating. If a girl is not mature enough within herself to solve differences without heated arguments—almost bordering on violence—she most likely should not even be dating. Problems must be worked out within one's self before being brought to the other person involved. When this action is reversed, anger becomes violence.

The purpose of anger is to deliver an emotional message. Anger is normal, but some ways I've seen girls express anger are not normal. Hysteria is definitely not the way to express

Creative Dating 59

an emotional message. A guy cannot cope with a girl who blows her top by shouting, crying, and screaming at the top of her lungs. This scares a fellow and all he will want to do is escape from this entire situation. He feels that a girl who can carry on in such a hateful manner to him, must not sincerely like him deep down in her heart. Both his feelings and his image are wounded.

If you are the type of girl who acts before she thinks, practice taking the violence out by talking to the wall or another inanimate listener. I know a girl who takes out her anger by talking the problem over with her stuffed animals. She circles them around her on her bed and lets off her steam in that way. Then she is able to think more clearly and be sensible about her problem. When you go to a person with a problem, make sure you have it worked out within yourself first.

Timing is so important too! The phone is not the time or place to discuss serious arguments. Statements are too often taken the wrong way and many arguments end with one or the other hanging up. This allows time to elapse and the problem grows even more out of proportion.

Bringing up a subject of disagreement when your guy is already downhearted is not appropriate either. Just after he's failed an important exam, or missed a vital play in a ball game is not correct timing. At this time he needs his ego put back together and spirits lifted. He doesn't need more burdens added to his heavy load!

When you bring up disagreements in a sweet, noncondemning way, your guy will be ready and willing to admit defeat. The least you can do is forgive him 100 percent. Forgiveness includes forgetting. Don't be guilty of telling him, "I forgive you," then the next time something comes up, putting the disagreement before him again. This is not true forgiveness. You need to forget the whole incident even occurred. God commanded Peter to forgive seventy times seven. (*See* Matthew 18:22.) Can we do less?

Maybe your guy isn't the type who brings up the subject first, or who likes to get things out in the open. If not, take the initiative yourself. Make the first move by telling him, "Something has been bothering me and I really would feel better if we discussed the matter." When you are in the wrong, don't hesitate to admit it. But, I learned that admitting your faults to a man is not degrading or dehumanizing. Rob respected me more when I began to learn to say, "I'm sorry." I need to say those meaningful words daily.

When you admit defeats, your guy does not think less of you, nor about how many faults you have. Instead it brings out his masculine urge to shelter and reassure you. He'll want to cuddle and assure you that you are still wonderful to him even with such a failure. No one appreciates people who claim to be perfect and never wrong. Just admit to your guy, "I was so wrong, I just can't handle such big things anyway." He will see the need for him to be there for you to rely on; he will then *want* to be there.

Childlike Reactions

Have you ever noticed that somehow children get away with acting just as they wish, yet they seem to fit in anywhere? Whenever you are stuck in a situation—not knowing just how to react—think of how a child would cope with the circumstance. Children just let their emotions shine through in all honesty; there's nothing fake about them. Here are some problem situations that girls have come to me with, because they were puzzled as to how to react.

TEASING When a guy teases, he is usually showing affection or flirting in his own little way. Don't be too sensitive to teasing; really it is a compliment. If you get overly embarrassed while being teased, or if the teasing is taking place in front of others, take action like a child. Stamp your foot and say, "I am not," or, "Well, I can't help it." These comments are much better accepted than sulking and being too hurt. Teasing isn't meant to cut deep down, but only to emphasize some cute little action you've done or characteristic you have.

MONOPOLIZING You and your guy need activities both alone and together. Some guys will try to go so "steadily" that they may as well be married. This is not good for either party of the dating couple. Separate times are both fun and needed. Having activities while apart makes the times together more appreciated and meaningful. If your fellow never goes out with "just the guys," then suggest a sport for him to become involved in. Then similarly, you should go out with "just the girls" either shopping or to slumber parties or perhaps join a girls' sports team at school or church. These times of being separated will be great conversation topics for when you are together. Also, you may not always be dating this one same boy. Consider the loneliness after breaking up, if you had no girl friends to fall back on. No couple should ever seclude themselves from the rest of the world and just be to themselves. We all need a variety of friends—and *lots* of them.

EMBARRASSMENTS The time will come when teasing gets carried a little too far and the time becomes embarrassing. The best way to react is in a shy, demure way. Don't try to talk or laugh your way out of the situation. I have been present to see girls embarrassed by their boyfriends absolutely to tears. If he gets this carried away, still be shy at the time, but definitely bring up the incident later. Explain to him that you feel you weren't being too sensitive about this, but that you were hurt to the point of harsh embarrassment.

He'll understand, and more importantly will learn from the lesson.

IGNORED When a guy ignores his date or girl friend, there *is* a reason. The reason could be that he needs a quiet time to think something out within himself. He usually just needs to be alone. Be understanding in the matter by not taking his withdrawal personally. If such ignoring continues, let him know that you crave his attention and it means a lot to you when he does pay attention. When he realizes you need him so badly, he'll come on stronger with consideration of you.

COMPLIMENTS Guys like to compliment their girl friends with words and with gifts. This, however, is not easy for some fellows to become accustomed to doing. Yet many girls don't encourage their fellows to compliment them simply by the way they react to complimentary words. (Admit it! We all do enjoy compliments!) I've seen a boy tell his gal how cute she looks in a certain outfit, and she answers, "Oh, I don't either. I look fat!" Or I've heard a boy say how good a girl looks with a certain hairstyle and she'll reply, "No, I don't! It's a mess!" Girls who repeatedly answer compliments with such negative replies will soon convince people that they're right. Pretty soon their fellow will begin to think, "Yes, she does look kinda fat"; or, "You know, her hair is always a mess." A simple, demure "Thank you" is all the answer a compliment requires. With the way that we gals like to receive compliments from our guys, there's no sense in hindering him from handing them out.

Asking and Receiving

When a boy gives you a gift, his only reward is seeing how pleased you are. Many fellows don't give because they receive no joy in their giving. Girls nowadays seem to have forgotten how to say the simple phrase "Thank you." If you have been ungrateful or unappreciative, it's no wonder your man doesn't shower you with presents.

Your guy wants to fulfill your desires and know he is pleasing you in doing so. Appreciation is communicated by words, attitude, and actions. Sincere gratitude shines through from a grateful heart.

Express your appreciation to your guy for the little things that he does—not for just the gifts he presents to you. Thank him for the little things in life, and he'll begin to give you those extras that you want. Thank him for the dates he escorts you on. Thank him for his thoughtfulness and politeness. Thank him for his being on time and for the nice way he treats your family. These expressions of gratitude will stir his feeling toward meeting your every need.

The biblical admonition, "It is more blessed to give than to receive," is so true. Your fellow has an emotional need of giving to fulfill. When you want something in particular, never demand or nag. Don't hint around either. He is not a mind reader. Trying to justify a desire or convince him will only make him feel guilty.

Perhaps your guy will ask what you would like for a particular special occasion. Be honest and direct. Just as a child asks her daddy for an ice-cream cone, tell him your desire. This will put him in the "King" position of being the only one who can fulfill your desires.

Be very appreciative of whatever gift he offers, whether it be one rose or a mink coat. Be surprised, elated, and excited as you receive his gift. He will want to do more and more for you just to see your pleasurable, girlish reaction.

Homework 3

1. Be a "Yes, let's" gal! Be enthusiastic about your boyfriend's ideas and suggestions.

2. Create a fun, exciting, original date for you and your guy. Let him know only the necessary essentials beforehand and surprise him with a date full of imagination.

3. Compliment him (your fellow) daily. Admire his virtues, his body, and his way of treating you.

4. Surprise your guy with a little gift. It could be something useful or something cute and humorous.

4

Dating Seriously

One of the young men whom you date may eventually become your lifetime companion and the father of your children. Set your goals high when choosing fellows to be interested in, since each one is a prospective husband. Don't make the mistake of agreeing to go out with a boy who has a bad reputation because you say it will be for "one simple date." A girl rarely knows if she will get serious with someone before the first date. You may get yourself involved and serious while just "casually dating."

Marriage Material—Him

Once you have in mind the qualities you want in a man, never settle for second-best. It may take a few dates for you to realize that the guy just does not have these qualities. When you are sure that there is no future in your relationship, it is not fair to him or to you to continue dating, just to have dates.

Use judgment in selecting a man suitable for a mate. If you are considering one who is lazy, dishonest, or of weak character, you are treading on dangerous ground. I've known girls who have allowed themselves to be charmed by men, only to find heartbreak in later life.

One of my main considerations when I was dating in college was, "Can I be truly proud of him?" I made it a point not to date anyone with whom I would be ashamed to walk into a crowded place. If I was asked out by a boy in whom I had no interest, I would arrange to have "previous plans." Turning down a guy is never wrong, provided you are polite and sincere. Fellows would rather never start a relationship than be hurt later. When you date steadily, you and he automatically are pegged together as a couple. If he has areas that you are ashamed of, you will be classified as having those same weak qualities. Be aware of character traits, masculinity, skills, and attitudes. If you can't be proud of his looks, voice, and even dress—then he's not *"the* one" for you.

You cannot hope to remake a guy into some preconceived image you may have in your mind. You must accept him exactly as he is. Not only will your efforts to change him be fruitless, but a barrier will grow between you when he realizes what you are trying to do. A number of girls claim, "But he *will* change." Don't tie a guy down by forcing him to make promises to drop certain bad habits or reach certain goals. These promises are unfair, because men need to be free. As he is now, could you always be happy with him? This is the thought to consider because changes just do not occur.

Watch the way your guy treats his family, especially his mother. This is the way he will someday treat his own household. Family similarity is important to consider. Background plays an important part in character, habits, and standards. Does your fellow take the lead in small circumstances now? If he isn't able to do so in dating, he won't be a strong leader in providing for his family later. The way he treats you now is a prediction of how he will treat you in marriage. If he doesn't open doors, send flowers, and offer masculine assistance now, don't expect such tender expressions of thoughtfulness in marriage. These inner qualities outweigh appearance and popularity, and so forth. Love that lasts is based on character, not sex appeal.

Be certain the one you consider marrying is a born-again Christian. You are only fooling yourself by thinking he will accept Christ later. The Scripture says, "Be ye not unequally yoked together . . ." (2 Corinthians 6:14). This goes for dating as well as marriage.

Although we should have aims and values by which we expect our guy to measure up, one cannot be unrealistic. No man is without flaw, faults, and even failures. Be guided—but not blinded—by your goals and expectations.

G-I-R-L

All through the day while playing, my little girl Missy mumbles to herself and her toys. Many times she gets frustrated when trying to convey a message to me in her little jumbled way because I don't correctly respond to her pleas. "Is it a toy she wants?" "Is she tired or hungry?" Sometimes I feel at a loss as to what to do for her because of our language barriers.

This is how most girls feel after hearing ideas and philosophies from parents, school, and religious groups. Every group claims to have the "truth" yet they all contradict each other. Some are good enough to live by—but not good enough to die by. The search is endless for many girls because they just don't know which way to turn.

Trying to "do good" isn't enough. No matter how many good deeds one does, something is still lacking inside. Ephesians 2:9 says, "Not of works, lest any man should boast." There has to be something, Someone more—a greater source than ourselves.

Parents don't often offer the answers, mostly because they honestly don't have the answers. Many teens are bitter towards their parents for not caring enough to show them the way to fill this void in their lives. Parents' hypocrisy and inconsistency cause hostility. Parents often don't practice what they preach. If your mom and dad fall into this category, don't let hostility take hold. They are possibly searching for truth just as hard as you are. I've seen many teens find Christ as their Saviour and, in turn, lead their whole family to Him. Just because your parents don't take the first step is no excuse for you not finding the Way.

The word *girl* spells it all out for you! Take a look at the word with me—letter by letter. *You* can be what these letters spell out. You *can* be total, complete, fulfilled through Christ.

G This first letter represents the initial step in finding the answer to many of your questions. First Timothy 6:6 says that ". . . godliness with contentment is great gain." There is no way that you can have this godly contentment spoken of here without first accepting Jesus Christ as your personal Saviour.

God sent His Son to die on the cross in payment for our sins. Jesus was the sacrifice for our sins. Ephesians 2:8 and 9 says, "For by grace are ye saved through faith; and that not of yourselves: it is the gift of God. Not of works, lest any man should boast." It's a *gift!* Your boyfriend could buy you a necklace for your birthday, but it wouldn't become yours until you actually reached out and took it. This is how it is with God's gift of eternal life. For it to become yours, you must receive it.

If you have never reached out to Him and accepted Jesus Christ as your personal Saviour, now is the time. Don't wait or put it off. He wants to come into your life and live through you because He loves you so much. I never experienced real joy until I finally gave my whole life and self to Jesus Christ, and let Him take control. You can have godliness, but not through your own strength. Ask Christ to come into your heart, forgive your sins, and give you eternal life. He alone will give you the courage and strength you need to face each day and to truly be a TOTAL GIRL.

I As a girl, you have a great *influence* on the people around you—more than you may realize. You influence your girl friends by the way you dress and act. They will pick up your actions and way of dress because teenagers are known for following their companions' ways. You follow the patterns your friends set concerning habits, dress, and places they go.

When considering this responsibility, examine the influence you personally are setting for others. Do you lead them to the right places? Is your example of dress and language a good one to follow? You may think, "But no one looks to me for inspiration." Don't fool yourself! Even when you are unaware, your influence is rubbing off onto someone you know. I've known so many girls who have younger sisters and have set a poor example for them to follow.

What about your influence on dates with guys? Does a Christlike testimony shine through or do you influence him in ways that could lead to trouble? You, the girl, set the atmosphere on your dates. If you get in the car and snuggle up close right from the start, what kind of influence is that on him? It tells him, "This is just a start," and encourages him further—perhaps to a situation neither of you can handle.

Because of Christ, you can set the right influence on others. With Him controlling your life you have the power to bring out the best in others and even influence them to accept Jesus as their Saviour, too! When your friends see the joy and peace He has given you, they will want what you have. What a responsibility! We have the power to influence the eternal destiny of our own friends! If we fail to show them the way to the Lord through our lives, they may never know until it is too late.

R When I tell you what the letter *R* stands for, you will probably think you can never be this. When a person accepts Christ and becomes a child of God, he becomes very *rich*. But, you say, you only get a two-dollar-a-week allowance! The Bible speaks of riches we obtain, but not in a monetary sense.

Proverbs 10:22 says, "The blessing of the Lord, it maketh rich...." My husband and I have very little as far as material pleasures of this life are concerned. Being in full-time Christian service, we probably never will. But, that certainly doesn't discourage or defeat us. We consider ourselves wealthy in the things of the Lord. He has blessed us bountifully and continues to bless daily.

You, as a Christian, have the same blessings. God's promises include a heavenly home, rewards, and His ever-present help in time of need. See if you don't find yourself counting blessings beyond your own belief. Our trouble as humans is that many times we just don't sit down and count them.

Some Christians have their priorities in the wrong perspective. They are so busy making a living to gain material goods that they let the important eternal riches slip by. I know Christians who have lived their own lives for years and finally (usually urged on by a tragic incident) started living for the Lord. They regret so much having wasted years on themselves after seeing how God does bless when we're in His perfect will. Don't let rich blessings pass you by while living for yourself. It doesn't pay off, because all earthly things quickly pass. Only what's done for Christ will last.

L This letter sums it all up. It completes the word *girl* as well as compiles all the qualities a fellow wants into one. It

Dating Seriously

is up to you, yourself, how *lovely* you will be before guys and before God.

From the very beginning we learned not to worry if we were not blessed naturally with striking beauty. Make the most of your best points! This is true inwardly as well as outwardly. How lovely are you inside the real you? Are your thoughts pure or full of filth and vanity? Do you go to places that can only lead to trouble and a bad reputation?

Only you can honestly answer these questions. Would you be embarrassed if everyone knew your secret thoughts, words, and deeds? God does know, girls. He looks on the heart, not on the outward appearance. When you think you are fooling everyone, don't kid yourself. God sees and knows and someday we will all be accountable unto Him.

In 2 Samuel 1:23 God speaks of being "lovely and pleasant" in our lives. This needs to apply to every aspect—the nicest we can look on the outside and the most honest and pure we can keep ourselves on the inside. This all really takes God's help! Our sinful nature keeps us slipping back if we try cleaning up our hearts by ourselves.

Daily devotions of reading a passage in the Bible and asking for God's help are essential. Whenever I fail to pause at the start of a day to ask for God's guidance and strength, my day goes miserably. I find myself blowing it all day! But, when I seek His help, He gives it to me and my day runs smoothly. Just knowing His Presence is with me enables me to face each new day with confidence. It's not hard, then, to have a smile on my face and a spring in my step. You can too; start each day with the Lord and see what a difference He makes.

You may have been in a crowded football stadium or in a large group of people and thought, "There are so many millions of people in this world, is there really one special guy just for me?" "How will I know him when I meet him?" "How long will I have to wait for him?"

Patience is a virtue we all have to ask the Lord for in abundance. However long the time drags on that you have to wait for your special guy, stick it out. Too many marriages have faltered after a girl accepted a proposal on the basis of thinking, "This is my last chance." Set your goal high and never settle for second best. ". . . wait patiently for him . . ." (Psalms 37:7). "Wait on the Lord: be of good courage, and he shall strengthen thine heart: wait, I say, on the Lord (Psalms 27:14).

Meanwhile, don't sit around feeling sorry for yourself. Pray daily for whomever the Lord has chosen as mate for you. He's out there somewhere and needs your prayerful support even now. God is shaping both of your lives in preparation for that day when you shall come together in precious realization of one another. Continue to better yourself, stay involved in many activities, and volunteer yourself in church and charitable organizations. Helping others will keep you unselfishly involved instead of wrapped up in self-pity.

Challenge yourself to memorize the Thirty-first Chapter of Proverbs. Then trust the Lord to help you to be this kind of woman. Keep these goals constantly before you and strive to be this virtuous woman whose priceless value is far above rubies.

Homework 4

1. Set some long-term goals for yourself—goals to be reached throughout your lifetime into marriage.

2. Read John 3. This free gift of salvation is yours for the asking.

3. When you have good rapport with your boyfriend, ask him to write down your three main weaknesses. Thank him—don't be offended—then work on these points.

4. Put into practice each day the concepts of being a TOTAL GIRL.

The Ten Qualities of True Love

1. True love is responsive totally to the other partner.
2. True love shows esteem and respect toward the partner.
3. True love always wants to give.
4. True love embraces a willingness to accept responsibility.
5. True love is marked with joy in the partner's presence and pain in his or her absence.
6. True love finds enjoyment without the need of physical expression.
7. True love has a protective attitude.
8. True love has the feeling of belonging.
9. True love is based on the common grounds of understanding.
10. True love looks to Christ for help and growth.

5

How to Measure the Quality of Your Love

Perhaps one of the most perplexing questions that has ever been raised is, "How will I know when I'm in love?" Do skyrockets zoom across the sky? Does a little cupid shoot an arrow into your heart? Will you lose your appetite or become constantly hungry?

For nine months I listened to my boyfriend (future husband) say those precious three words without replying them back to him. I just had to be sure—but how? How was Rob *so* certain that he loved me? I wanted to be equally as confident, but could not find the formula in books or experienced friends. Rob was so patient while I was sorting out my feelings. He never once tried to pry the phrase out of me.

One Sunday afternoon while we were alone on a picnic, I shocked my own ears by listening to myself say, "Rob, I love you." I had not planned to tell him that day—I just blurted it out. I couldn't stop saying it over and over. That's when I knew I was in love. I had to quit trying to reason out my feelings. I tried to be too logical instead of just letting my heart do the talking.

This final section is going to assume that you, as a TOTAL GIRL, have progressed through the previously outlined stages of being what a guy desires and finding your man. Now, hold on! Don't become discouraged if you aren't one of the few to whom this section applies appropriately at this time. Read on—you will pleasantly find yourself needing this information, and possibly sooner than you dreamed. These ten checkpoints are valuable to you now, if you are presently involved in a serious relationship with your boyfriend. The checkpoints are even more beneficial to the gals who have not yet entered into a serious relationship. When that special guy comes along, you will have the advantage of being able to check your feelings all along as they grow and develop.

1. True Love Is Responsive Totally to the Other Partner.

When you truly love someone, you will totally accept him just as he is. Many girls fall "in love" with a handsome face or great body build instead of the person inside that body. Girls, you will come closer to that happy-ever-after ending if you marry a person, not a body.

One starry-eyed couple repeated the marriage vows and anxiously set out for a memorable honeymoon. After arriving at their motel suite, the bride began her bedtime preparations. A very shocked groom sat by watching as she removed the flowing blond wig, curly eyelashes, and restraining girdle. Had this fellow married the young lady solely for appearance, he was to be extremely disappointed. What would he have left after finding out how "deceived" he had been all during their courtship? We gals need to have more to offer than a few false pretenses of beauty.

Equally so, your future groom *will* disappoint you in marriage—if you base your "love" on bulging biceps and broad shoulders. You will want to be proud of your man's physical appearance—true; however his high points must be deeper than the surface. What will you have in a mate in a few years when his physical attractiveness begins deteriorating? His skin will show age wrinkles, those muscles are going to weaken, and that flowing hair you so admire will begin to vanish into thin air!

Ask yourself this important question: "Would there be enough to love if all those physical changes took place?" Could you still look him in the eyes (they may even require glasses) and say, "I love you even more than the day I met you"? Don't laugh—such changes are bound to take place. You are going to want—and even expect—your husband to love you more as the anniversaries pass by. You won't want him to begin looking elsewhere just because your waistline bulges a bit after childbirth, or your glowing complexion requires a little more makeup than before.

Our society has become so sex-oriented that marriage is played up to be one big continued sex party. Living with someone facing life's everyday pressures can not always be described as a party. Only fairy-tale couples live that way. One sure way to be disappointed in marriage is to go into the relationship imagining pure bliss all the time.

Being responsive totally to your partner involves some lifetime commitments. You will be committing yourself in marriage, restricting nothing. No matter if his hair does fall out, or his stomach does get a spare tire, your commitments should stand firm with him. This is why marriages based on physical attractiveness do not flourish. Now true love remains totally responsive through any changes. Check your feelings toward your guy by watching to see if they fluctuate from day to day. If he doesn't look as sharp at times, do you feel less like being affectionate and personable toward him? Remember, when he comes home from a construction job, he won't look or smell too appealing. But, he will need you there for praise and encouragement just the same. And no one looks perfectly presentable when they first awake in the morning. Does this mean you aren't going to have anything to do with him until he has showered and shaved?

I'm not saying that every good-looking guy has no qualities deep on the inside. Nor do I advocate you marrying someone whose appearance you would be ashamed of. But, keep your priorities in the right perspective, putting major emphasis on a man's inner character. Make sure it is one you can respect, honor, and cherish for all of time.

2. True Love Shows Esteem and Respect Toward the Partner.

This statement reflects not only the person's attitude, but also his actions toward the partner in a relationship. This is important throughout the dating period as well as in marriage.

True love puts the other person on a pedestal. Such esteem for your mate does not mean that you will not realize he has faults and disabilities. However, this type of respect allows you to understand that he is human—but is the nearest thing to a King in your eyes. When others first meet your fellow, they may not see what you see in him. But after a while, they will be conformed to your way of thinking by your attitude of admiration for him.

I remember baby-sitting for a family with three girls when I was a teenager. I knew the girls' mother, but had never met the father of the home. But, I sure felt like I knew him! Through the little girls' conversation and actions I learned about a man whom I gradually pictured in my mind as being close to perfect. These girls were constantly making their daddy little presents, cooking special goodies for him, and doing their chores readily so their daddy would be proud. "What kind of a superdaddy and husband must this be?" I wondered.

Then one evening I was finally to meet him! I couldn't keep myself from peeking out the front window to watch the three girls excitedly run down the sidewalk as their daddy's car drove into the driveway. What a surprise met my eyes! I had this man's image pictured so differently. A very common, rather short, plain-clothed man stepped out of the car. He huddled all of the girls into his arms at one time, answering their requests for kisses and candy. Just meeting this man on the street, one would not be impressed. But, his wife had set these little girls the right example. She had shown them that this man was the King of their house who had final control. He was to be served, obeyed, and respected. Because this mother had the right idea, these girls would have no role conflicts in their future marriages.

It just makes me burn inside every time I hear a husband or a child say they are going home to the "ol' lady." Such references show great lack of respect, and make one wonder if love is even in the home at all.

Anything that causes one to lose respect for the other person is not real love. For example, true love does not find the partners constantly pawing all over each other. True love does not try to convince you to let things happen that you will regret later. You see, girls, when a guy truly loves you, he would not ask you to let him do something that would hurt you. This includes you as a person, your body, and your reputation.

Here is where many fellows have a double standard. Such a guy wants a girl who can give him a hot Saturday-night date, but when it comes to settling down—that's a different story. The girl such a guy looks for then must have different qualities. This type—who has two standards for the girls he wants—is worthless to the girl who is honestly searching for the right kind of man. Oh, sure, he will try to sweet-talk you into believing that yielding to his desires proves that you return his "love." But after such a guy has enjoyed a cheap fling for a while, he will look elsewhere for a permanent relationship.

Many a girl is badly hurt inside after such a letdown. Here all the while she is made to believe that the fellow is leading her into a serious engagement. Then the girl is put through the embarrassment and heartbreak of terminating the relationship. All she has to show is her broken heart and memories of false belief. Some girls have more than that to show. It is when shattered self-pride, or even an unborn baby is involved, that the situation is extremely severe emotionally for a girl. Time after time, a guy will lead his so-called girl friend on too far by saying that if she does not yield, she doesn't care for him as he does for her. After he finds out the consequences of a probable pregnancy, he skips out. I know girls who have been left to face the nine months of adjustment in loneliness. Then there is the girl who hears from the father of their child only by receiving a check to cover childbirth costs. As if that mended the broken heart, or lessened the pain!

Girls, you never know if a guy is going to marry you until those vows are actually spoken. Anything could happen even in those last few days—from his reneging to a tragic car accident. You need to have respect for your husband when you marry him—and he for you—not guilt feelings after taking advantage of each other before marriage for a few moments of pleasure. To be able to respect and submit to your husband as the Bible teaches, you must respect him as a person first.

3. True Love Always Wants to Give.

Many people enter into marriage thinking, "What's in this for me?" In a relationship where each partner needs to be giving his complete 100 percent, there is no room for such thinking. Instead of saying, "Will this guy make me happy all the rest of my life?" you must ask yourself the question, "Can I make this guy happy for the rest of his life?"

Marriage nowadays is built so much on giving to self. The girl marries because *she* wants to be in her own home, have her own children, and get away from her parents. Men marry because they feel this is the thing that will make them feel worthwhile and self-sufficient.

When anyone marries for any reason other than to bring joy and fulfillment to the one they love, the marriage already has one foot in the divorce court. How true is the phrase "Give and it shall be given unto you." The only trouble with most of us is that we want the rewards of giving too soon.

Many marriage partners have the philosophy that "I did such and such for him, now he should do something for me." This is not the way payday for good deeds works! We're not to go around expecting or anticipating rewards for some little something we did for our mates. Love gives—expecting nothing in return.

I enjoy sending anonymous cards with thoughts of love or appreciation to people who mean something special to me. Usually these recipients never know that it was I who sent them. But, I know their day was brightened because of a little expression of thoughtfulness. That's my reward!

This is the way giving in marriage needs to be. The other person's desires must come before your own. Sometimes this means great sacrifices. It may require you to rearrange your entire scheduling for some spur of the moment whim that your husband dreams up. It means smiling when he spends the entire paycheck on something for the house when you had counted on buying a beautiful new winter coat.

Check your feelings—do you groan and hold a grudge when you have to go along with your boyfriend's wishes? Are you willing to sacrifice friends, places to go, and money for what he wants? True love takes pleasure in being able to give to the loved one—even if the demands seem great and rewards few.

4. True Love Embraces a Willingness to Accept Responsibility.

That statement explains the reason why I just cannot believe that couples that shack up together are really in love. These couples do not care to accept the responsibility of marriage, yet they expect to enjoy the pleasures that come with it. That kind of reasoning just does not work. It may sound great in theory, but when put into practice, it is not feasible. Eventually the couple living together will need the bond of marriage, or result in splitting up. I have never known such arrangements to last more than a few months.

Many folks say that during the next generation the institution of marriage is going to dissolve and become obsolete. I cannot believe such predictions in light of biblical principles. God ordained marriage, and as long as there are couples in love who also love God, there will be marriages. God knew this was the best way for man and woman to live together. Instead, mankind has to try his own methods to see if they work better than God's. We all know this is impossible.

Some couples enter marriage thinking, "Well, if this doesn't work out, then we can always get a divorce." What a sad thought to be thinking as you walk down the aisle! Anyone who has ever experienced a divorce or in the immediate family knows that it is not just a simple signing of a document. So many innocent lives are affected as the pain lags on indefinitely.

When you repeat the vow *I do,* you are, in effect, saying, "I will stick it out." Sometimes the going gets rough as making a truly great marriage takes a lot of work. Everything in marriage does not come readily, so keep in mind that it *will* take your 100 percent effort. When the going gets rough, remember Isaiah 43:2. In this precious verse God promises to be with us as we go through deep waters of difficulty and great trouble. *This* is why so many marriages fail. The couple forgets to turn to the Source of answers to all their problems. They read sex manuals and see marriage counselors, but fail to go to God's Word. No couple will ever feel like giving up after they have prayer together. While getting up off their knees, they will know their marriage has hope because God will help them.

Divorce has become too easy to obtain in our country. Don't let yourself be guilty of thinking that your marriage could ever end in divorce. If you even entertain such thoughts, then divorce will always be a possibility for cop-out in the back of your mind. Every time some little conflict arises you will begin to think, "Maybe we weren't meant for each other after all." Ask God to remove such thoughts—even now as you pray toward your eventual marriage.

True love gives the woman a willingness to take care of the home, and a man the desire to provide for the home. It used to always puzzle me how Christian housewives could go about their daily household tasks so cheerfully. That's what comes with true love—a desire to accept the responsibilities.

If you were hired as the secretary for a businessman, there would be specific duties you would be expected to handle. The same principle carries through marriage. Women who take no pride in the appearance of their home—or themselves—show no love toward their family or husband. Check your feelings by seeing if you are really willing to fulfill the duties as a wife for that guy for "as long as you both shall live."

5. True Love Is Marked With Joy in the Partner's Presence and Pain in His or Her Absence.

Throughout the year at college that Rob and I first began dating, we cherished every opportunity to see each other.

Classes, clubs, cheerleading, jobs and all the other campus activities made those times few and far between. I remember just living for those moments we would be able to spend together. When we were apart I would daydream about Rob and doodle his name all over class notes. I spent much of my time staring out my dorm window, in hopes of catching a glimpse of him across the campus.

Even now when Rob has to go to out-of-town engagements, I am almost lost without him. My whole day centers around his homecoming in the early evening. When he has to work late or be away in the evening, I miss his company and presence in the home so much.

This exemplifies a characteristic of love. Not that when your guy is away, you will worry continually about his actions or his feelings—not *that* kind of pain when he's not there. I have enough confidence in our love to know that if Rob were called away for two years of service, that when he returned to me, our love would even be stronger that the day he departed. The feeling of pain is due to the loss of companionship and security that his being there offers.

When you love someone, you will have joy being in his presence. Your like interests and complementing personalities will present new forms of enjoyment each time you are together. One girl was considering the possibility of marriage when she enrolled in the TOTAL GIRL classes. She was concerned about such a serious step because of the problem her boyfriend had of embarrassing her in front of their friends. He would tease and joke about her to the extent that she would beg him to leave parties early. Even though their private times were enjoyable together, this girl would never be happy in marriage. Instead of being proud to show off her mate, she would always have the fear of being embarrassed by him in front of a group.

Genuine love is always characterized by the good times

couples have while together, and the longing for the partner during separation. Do you enjoy having your boyfriend around—doing nothing special—just being together? Or are you rather relieved when he's gone so you can let down and be yourself for a while? Consider both of these attitudes when deciding if his presence brings joy, and his absence brings pain.

6. True Love Finds Enjoyment Without the Need of Physical Expression.

When a couple is sincerely in love they will find moments of pure happiness just by being with each other. Have you ever been on a date when you felt uncomfortable, unless either you or he were constantly talking? You had to keep one step ahead of him so that the conversation would not lag and silence prevail. In marriage, you and your mate would wear yourselves out physically and emotionally, if you had to constantly keep up that pace. There will be many evenings when you both, after an exhausting day, simply feel like relaxing together watching television. Have you ever taken notice of elderly folks as they sit together perhaps in a porch swing or rocking chairs? How peaceful and content they seem—just to know that their loved ones are nearby!

I guess this thought really hit me as Rob and I drove to our secluded honeymoon cottage. It was located on a lake, a two-hour drive from our wedding location. After all the hustle and bustle of a big church wedding and reception, we were both in need of the two-hour get-away drive. Driving along, I felt my body relax after the hectic year of preparation for that eventful day. A mutual understanding of our feelings communicated between the two of us as we traveled together in complete silence. I remember thinking, "I never knew we could be so content with each other."

A girl who has to have her guy pawing all over her every minute she's with him had better check her motives for dating him. Because a fellow is a good make-out does not automatically mean he is a good marriage prospect. You should not feel insecure if he doesn't constantly have his arm around you, or isn't always holding your hand. This is one sure way of telling if your relationship is mostly physical. Perhaps you should consider this possibility, if your boyfriend needs to constantly have some form of physical contact.

Certainly there is a time and a place for hand-holding and other meaningful signs of affection. Driving down the street in broad daylight, or stopped at a stoplight are absolutely not two of the most appropriate places. A guy has enough trouble handling the driving without you all but sitting in his lap, or laying your head across his chest. I always wonder about the couples who never cease to fondle each other. Usually this shows that all they care about is body attention. Seeing such outward displays of affection in public makes me really wonder what they must do in private!

Many girls actually like their boyfriend to cuddle them in front of people. This kind of girl feels that the display is showing others how much her guy really likes her. She wants her boyfriend to always be at her side, never allowing him to have a good time with others. Such possessiveness drives away fellows instead of making them more attached. Let your man show his affection for you by his manners, courtesy, and politeness toward you rather than constant physical attachment. You don't have to be concerned that others will not think he likes you, if he keeps his hands off of you. The message will come through, as he shows respect for you, instead of using your body as a play toy.

Just being together—that's the key to true love. Just because that guy is *who* he is, is reason enough to enjoy being in his presence. Beware if your relationship requires constant physical expression. Whether it's your idea or his, the priorities of your relationship need to change before marriage is considered.

7. True Love Has a Protective Attitude.

The female bear is a relatively calm animal, but let something threaten her cub's safety and she becomes a ferocious savage beast. A human being has the same protective instincts for the one he loves. If humanly possible, a mate will prevent any harm from coming to his or her partner.

Nothing is more discouraging than to hear something untasteful or critical being spoken about the one you love. Not only will this hurt you, but it will also make the protective instinct swell up inside you. You will want to stand up for the loved one who is being torn down. You should be able to trust the one who loves you to do the same. He should want to rush to your rescue when trouble threatens.

I'm thankful that I have this assurance in my husband. I can recall one incident where I really was in the wrong, but Rob stood by me and supported my actions. Then later, as we discussed the situation, I realized that I was wrong—and Rob knew it all the time. Yet, he did not join opposite sides in front of anyone which would have caused me embarrassment.

Not only should the one you love shield you from the criticism of others, he needs to bring up his gripes only in private. Just as a child is ashamed to receive a spanking in front of his friends, we must not voice faults of our loved ones in public. Your guy should praise and exalt you in front of others—not tear you down. If he feels you acted to giddy at a party, he should bring up the subject after you are away from the crowd. When he notices your slip showing, it would be appropriate to draw you aside to inform you of the problem—not right in front of everyone. Someone who truly loves a person will not make a spectacle of that person. He will, rather, talk about her best qualities and bring up the good points.

I never did go for the type of guy who is one big joker. I'm not a person who can take teasing very well; probably because most teasing usually ends up in true criticism. Do your boyfriend's jokes cut deep and hurt you? Too often this is how innocent joking ends up. First a joke is told about a dog with funny hair. Then the tale is related to your own hair, and before you know it, some very cutting remarks are made about the way your hair looks. There you sit with nowhere to turn, and everyone is making fun of the style, length, and color of your hair. That's when joking isn't too funny!

Criticisms can wear away at a relationship faster than anything else. Sarcastic remarks, even if they start out to be funny, will hurt in an unforgettable manner. Don't get into the habit of picking at the little things about the one you love. Pretty soon you will be concentrating so much on those petty faults, that you won't be able to see any good shining through.

If your boyfriend picks, teases, and criticizes now—your family ties will not be very strong. Eventually your children will pick up the same habit. If all they hear is Daddy cutting down Mommy, it will quickly soak in. They will lose respect for their mother because all they have ever heard are critical comments about her. This image obviously is wrong, and places confusion in children's minds.

It is true that "a friend in need is a friend indeed." This is how it is in true love—each will shield and protect the other. Such assurance in a relationship brings security and knowledge that you will never stand alone.

8. True Love Has the Feeling of Belonging.

Have you ever found yourself at a gathering and, even though you knew the people there, you still felt very "out of it"? I sure have—and it isn't a very comfortable feeling at all. When you fall in love, however, those feelings of insecurity will change into a deep sense of belonging. It will not matter where you are, who you are with, alone or in a crowd—the confidence that accompanies true love will comfort you. Your love doesn't even have to be right at your side for this peaceful assurance to accompany you—just the deep-down knowledge of your love is enough.

I remember the first week after Rob presented me with my engagement ring. Finally, our love was announced and public for the world to know! I just could not stop staring at that beautiful diamond! It seemed as though if I were to take my eyes off it, it might vanish from my finger. The reason I (and every other newly engaged girl) could not stop looking at that engagement ring, was not because of its delicate beauty. Rather, it was because of its meaning and what the symbol stands for. The significance of the ring symbolizes a unified love between two people. Every time I viewed my ring, I was reminded of the love that Rob and I shared. This gave me a sense of belonging and security that I had never before experienced.

It doesn't even take the viewing of a ring, necklace, or picture to know such security. When true love abounds, the feeling is automatic. It will just be there—no one can describe or define it. But, when it comes, *you will know*.

Security and the assurance of belonging are essential to the well-being of a girl. While guys are more independent, we girls have the need of knowing that we are secure in a relationship. A man has this need fulfilled through his occupational success, and by admiration of his manliness by a woman. Our security, however, has to be reinstated and assured to us almost daily. Without this assurance in your love, you will not be able to function properly and meet his needs as they arise. You will, instead, be too busy worrying and wondering about your own role in your relationship.

Both partners have to fulfill the other's needs equally. When one slacks off, he himself will suffer in the long run. This truth was clearly presented in the discussion about "filling his cup." When we gals fail to compliment and admire our men enough, we suffer by not receiving any overflow from them in return.

If your guy does not provide the security that you need—especially when contemplating marriage—consider the future carefully. You don't want to go through life wondering if your husband is going to come home at night, worrying if he is going to provide financially, or feeling insecure because of the lack of assurance of his love. There will be hard times that arise; but the faith and trust in your love which gives security will see you through.

9. True Love Is Based on the Common Grounds of Understanding.

What was it that first attracted you to your one special guy? Was it his appearance—his voice—his manners? Thinking back, I'm sure you recall something unique about that special fellow that caught your attention and turned your eye in his direction. When you began dating, you surely found more about him that pleased you. The dating period is a time to discover interests that both partners have in common.

Couples that really hope to make a go of their relationship must have more in common than both liking to eat pizza. After all, how much conversation can be built around the subject of pizza? Plus, a person can only eat pizza just so long! I realize that is extreme, but when it comes right down to it, it's a shame that many couples have just about that much in common.

With some couples, the only common interest they share is physical attraction. Much of the time they spend together is not even enjoyed unless they are pawing all over each other. This weak relationship would really suffer in marriage. The poor couple would have nothing to share together, until they got in bed that night. "But," you may argue, "all young couples dwell heavily on physical attraction. The rest comes after marriage." Not true. Marriage is a bigger step than most young couples realize. There are many immediate adjustments. If the relationship is not strong in all areas *before* marriage, it will not hold up under the initial marital strains. Decisions about finances, a family, in-laws, and the home itself are very pressing after the honeymoon. If all the couple has to fall back on is a handful of kisses—the marriage is off to a weak start.

I'm not saying that you should *not* enjoy the way your future husband shows his affection toward you. After all, he's going to be the only man you'll be kissing for the rest of your life. It is just so important to keep priorities in their right perspective.

Not only are common grounds of interest important, agreement on important convictions is also essential. Religious and moral convictions need to be discussed, and the standards set *before marriage*. There have been many couples who honestly love one another—but have split up. They just could not cope with conflicting convictions. Had these been decided before marriage, the suffering would not have had to take place.

Being agreed on common grounds early in a relationship will save a lot of heartache when it comes to raising a family, too. Children must not see conflicts between their parents, or they will become confused and insecure. This is especially important when it comes to disciplining the children. If children know one parent is more apt to give in, they will always go to that one, and become resentful toward the stern parent.

The key to having common grounds of understanding in your relationship with a guy is for *you* to set your standards early; then settle only for a man who is equally convicted. If you compromise because you want the guy so badly, regrets and conflicts are bound to appear later. True love is in agreement; true love is *not* based on confusion and conflict.

10. True Love Looks to Christ for Help and Growth.

Love that remains strong enough for a lasting marriage can only come from above. It is only fitting, then, that couples go to Jesus Christ when problems arise. By doing this they will grow spiritually together.

Everyone needs to be faithful in having regular, individual, personal Bible study and prayer. In addition—as often as possible—the family needs to gather together around God's Word. Even if it is only you and your husband, this precious time of sweet communion can stabilize your marriage as nothing else can. A relationship is not going to continue at one rate. The love will either grow stronger or get weaker. To help your marriage get off to a good start, this pattern of having devotions together needs to be set early while dating.

The trials that come along the way will not hit nearly so hard if the couple is accustomed to praying together. When trouble does arise, it will be the most natural thing in the world for them to go to the Lord in prayer. After all, God gave us this love in the first place. The least we can do in return is turn it back over to Him to be used for His honor and glory!

Conclusion

TOTAL GIRL: This is the Today Girl that you can become when you let go of your own self and let Christ live in and through you—Christ-centered, Christ-controlled. The Holy Spirit living in you will bring these qualities into your life as you yield fully to Him. God will then be able to complete the girl He created into a Total Woman—who will share a lifetime of love and happiness with her husband in a Spirit-filled home.

Exciting, isn't it!